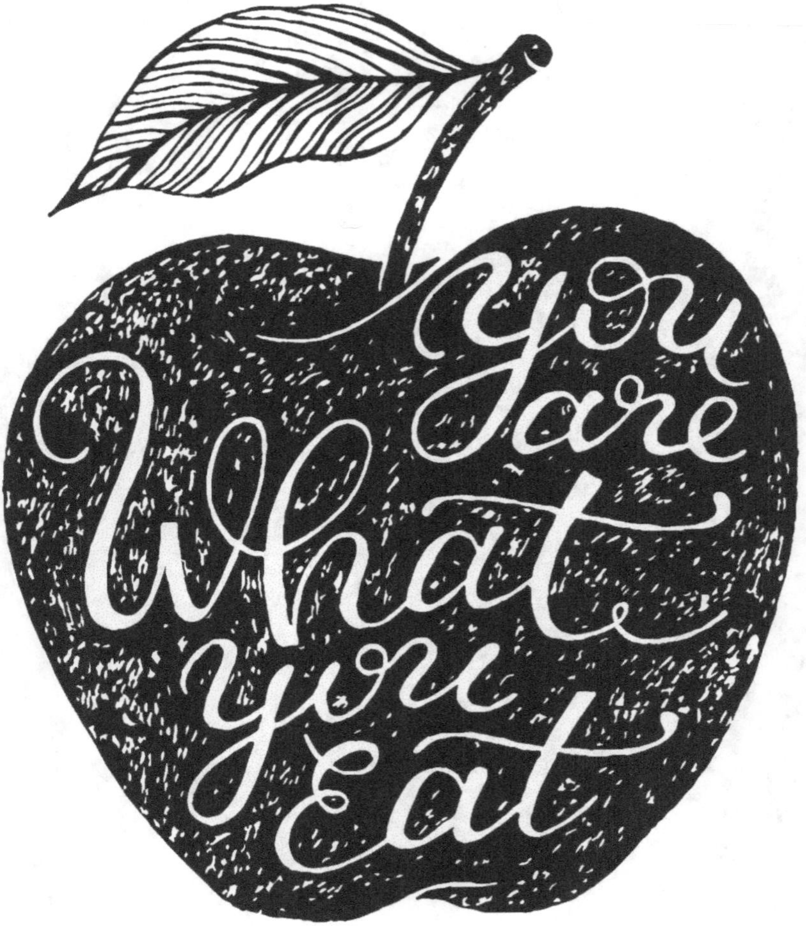

# 90 Day
# Daily Nutrition Tracker

Track your meals, exercise, sleep and hydration.
Set goals and check in with them weekly.
Stay inspired with regular doses of motivation!

# HOW TO USE THIS BOOK

Whether you are trying to lose weight, gain weight, improve your food choices or just track what you are eating, drinking and how you are moving, this 90-day daily nutrition tracker will help keep you on task.

## Page 1 - Start Where You Are
Take stock of where you are now.  Write down your current weight and measurements, and any other stats that you want to track.

## Page 2 - Set Your Goals
Start by thinking about what you hope to achieve and writing it down. Putting pen to paper will help you clarify your goals and make them more real and motivating.

## Page 3 - Healthy New Habits
Turn a new behavior into a habit! Track 4 new habits over the full 90 days, or work on smaller habits in 30 day chunks.

## Page 5 - Don't Break the Chain
Gain a sense of accomplishment for every day you complete the nutrition tracker. Don't break the chain!

## From Page 7 - Daily Pages
The daily pages provide space for what you eat and, if required, the calories / carbs / points consumed. Log your water consumption, fruit and veg intake and sleep. Did you exercise? What can you improve?  If it was a great day, make a note of the page number and add it to the Best Days section on page 122.

## From Page 14 - Weekly Check-in
Every 7 days you will want to check in to see how you are doing, and what you can improve over the next week.

## Page 121 - Final Check-in
You've worked hard for 90 days. How did you do?

## Page 122 - Best Days
For quick reference, keep an index of your best days.

## Page 123 - What Next?

# START WHERE YOU ARE

Date: _______________

Weight: _______________

Chest: _______________

Waist: _______________

Hips: _______________

Thigh: _______________

Calf: _______________

—— Fitness Assessment ——

_______________

_______________

_______________

_______________

_______________

_______________

_______________

_______________

How I'm feeling now:

Room for improvement:

A JOURNEY OF A THOUSAND MILES

## BEGINS

*With*

—— A SINGLE STEP ——

# SET YOUR GOALS

I will:

How:

It will make me feel:

Date: _______________________________

Weight: _____________________________

Chest: ______________________________

Waist: ______________________________

Hips: _______________________________

Thigh: ______________________________

Calf: _______________________________

———— Fitness Goals————

# HEALTHY NEW HABITS

Goal: _______________________________

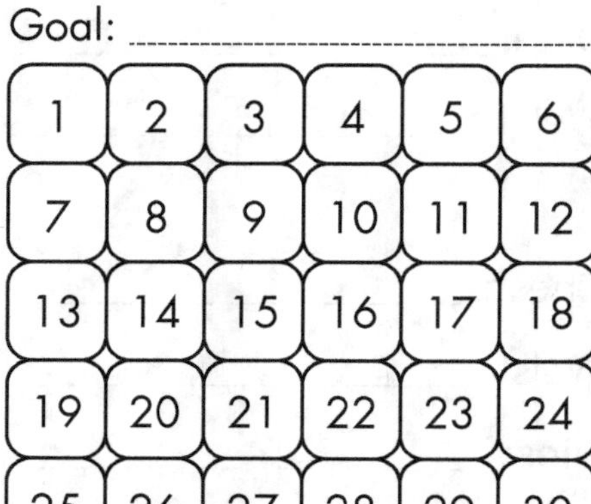

Goal: _______________________________

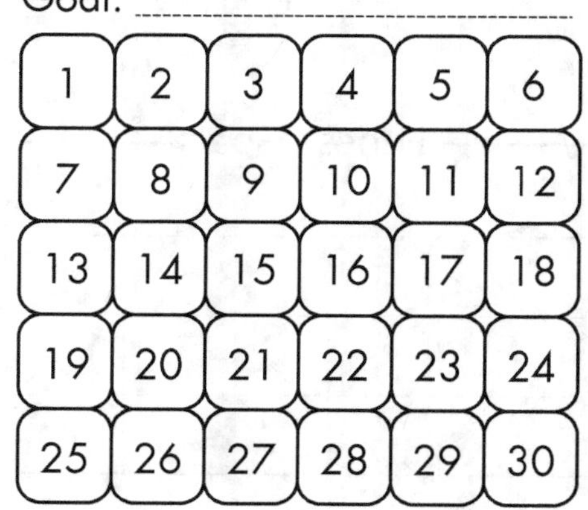

Goal: _______________________________

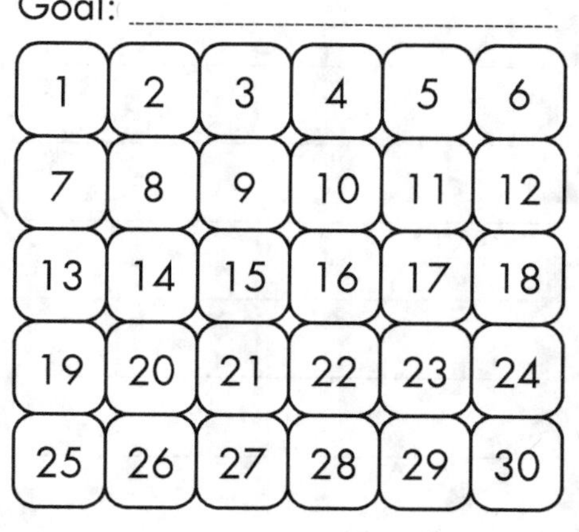

# HEALTHY NEW HABITS

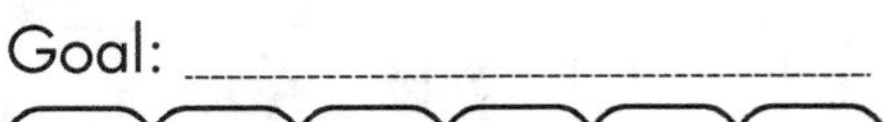

Goal: _______________________________

| 1 | 2 | 3 | 4 | 5 | 6 |
| 7 | 8 | 9 | 10 | 11 | 12 |
| 13 | 14 | 15 | 16 | 17 | 18 |
| 19 | 20 | 21 | 22 | 23 | 24 |
| 25 | 26 | 27 | 28 | 29 | 30 |

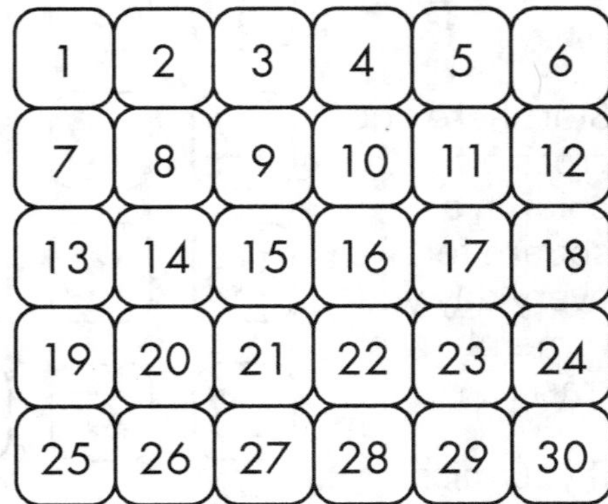

Goal: _______________________________

| 1 | 2 | 3 | 4 | 5 | 6 |
| 7 | 8 | 9 | 10 | 11 | 12 |
| 13 | 14 | 15 | 16 | 17 | 18 |
| 19 | 20 | 21 | 22 | 23 | 24 |
| 25 | 26 | 27 | 28 | 29 | 30 |

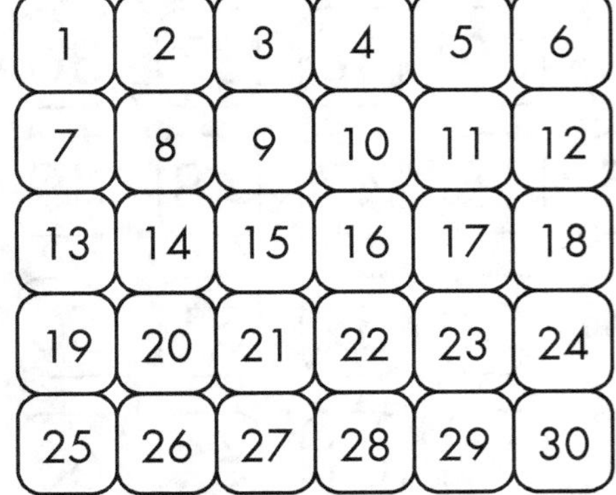

Goal: _______________________________

| 1 | 2 | 3 | 4 | 5 | 6 |
| 7 | 8 | 9 | 10 | 11 | 12 |
| 13 | 14 | 15 | 16 | 17 | 18 |
| 19 | 20 | 21 | 22 | 23 | 24 |
| 25 | 26 | 27 | 28 | 29 | 30 |

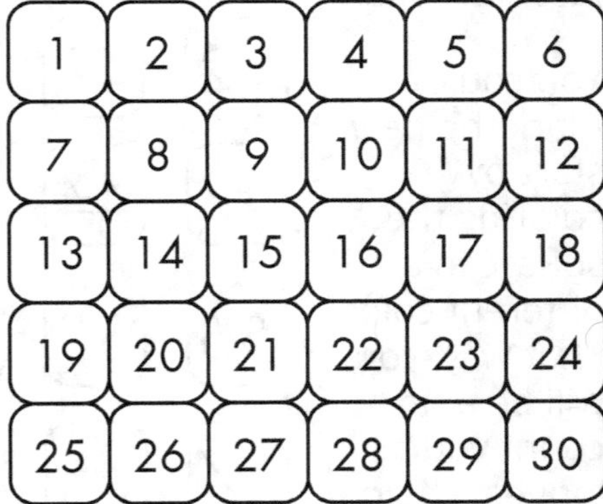

Goal: _______________________________

| 1 | 2 | 3 | 4 | 5 | 6 |
| 7 | 8 | 9 | 10 | 11 | 12 |
| 13 | 14 | 15 | 16 | 17 | 18 |
| 19 | 20 | 21 | 22 | 23 | 24 |
| 25 | 26 | 27 | 28 | 29 | 30 |

Goal: _______________________________

| 1 | 2 | 3 | 4 | 5 | 6 |
| 7 | 8 | 9 | 10 | 11 | 12 |
| 13 | 14 | 15 | 16 | 17 | 18 |
| 19 | 20 | 21 | 22 | 23 | 24 |
| 25 | 26 | 27 | 28 | 29 | 30 |

Goal: _______________________________

| 1 | 2 | 3 | 4 | 5 | 6 |
| 7 | 8 | 9 | 10 | 11 | 12 |
| 13 | 14 | 15 | 16 | 17 | 18 |
| 19 | 20 | 21 | 22 | 23 | 24 |
| 25 | 26 | 27 | 28 | 29 | 30 |

# DON'T BREAK THE CHAIN!

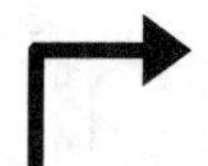

Start here and cross off or color in a square for every day you remember to track.

If you miss a day, don't beat yourself up! Just start again.

You could mark the new start by coloring the square in a different color. That way, you will be able to count your longest chain and challenge yourself to beat it!

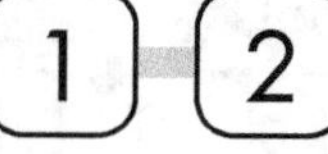

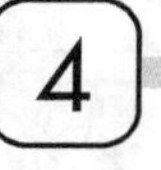

| 1 | 2 | 3 | 4 | 5 | 6 | 7 |
|---|---|---|---|---|---|---|
| 14 | 13 | 12 | 11 | 10 | 9 | 8 |
| 15 | 16 | 17 | 18 | 19 | 20 | 21 |
| 28 | 27 | 26 | 25 | 24 | 23 | 22 |
| 29 | 30 | 31 | 32 | 33 | 34 | 35 |
| 42 | 41 | 40 | 39 | 38 | 37 | 36 |
| 43 | 44 | 45 | 46 | 47 | 48 | 49 |
| 56 | 55 | 54 | 53 | 52 | 51 | 50 |
| 57 | 58 | 59 | 60 | 61 | 62 | 63 |
| 70 | 69 | 68 | 67 | 66 | 65 | 64 |
| 71 | 72 | 73 | 74 | 75 | 76 | 77 |
| 84 | 83 | 82 | 81 | 80 | 79 | 78 |
| 85 | 86 | 87 | 88 | 89 | 90 | |

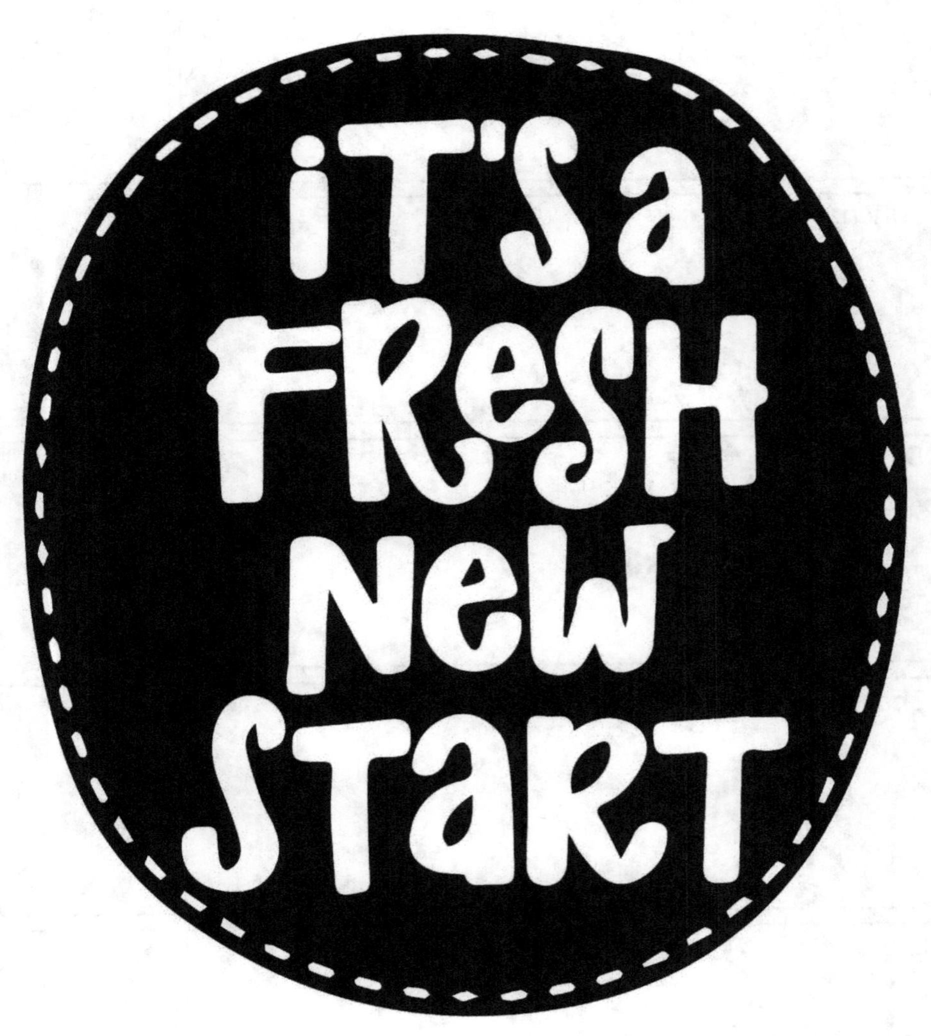

iT'S a
FReSH
NeW
StaRT

Breakfast:

Lunch:

Dinner:

Snacks and Drinks:

Exercise:

What went well? ________________________________________

What can I do better? ____________________________________

Breakfast:

Lunch:

Dinner:

Snacks and Drinks:

Exercise:

What went well? _______________________________________________

What can I do better? ___________________________________________

## DAY 03  DATE:

**Breakfast:**

**Lunch:**

**Dinner:**

**Snacks and Drinks:**

**Exercise:**

What went well? ______________________________________________________________

What can I do better? _________________________________________________________

# DAY 04  DATE:

Breakfast:

Lunch:

Dinner:

Snacks and Drinks:

Exercise:

What went well? _______________________________________________

What can I do better? __________________________________________

◀━━━━━ DAY 05  DATE:  ━━━━━▶

Breakfast:

Lunch:

Dinner:

Snacks and Drinks:

Exercise:

What went well? _______________________________________________

What can I do better? __________________________________________

Breakfast:

Lunch:

Dinner:

Snacks and Drinks:

Exercise:

What went well? _______________________________________________________

What can I do better? ___________________________________________________

◄──────── DAY 07  DATE:

Breakfast:

Lunch:

Dinner:

Snacks and Drinks:

Exercise:

What went well? _______________________________________________________

What can I do better? ___________________________________________________

# WEEKLY CHECK-IN

How have I done?

Any takeaways?

Date: _______________________________

Weight: _____________________________

—— Fitness Achievements ——

When you decide to cut back or give up a regular food or drink item, it can leave a void in your life. It is important to fill that void with something else that provides similar satisfaction but is better for you. Think about some of the voids you have felt this week or anticipate in the future, and come up with healthy substitution ideas.

Void: _________________ Substitution: _______________________

Void: _________________ Substitution: _______________________

Void: _________________ Substitution: _______________________

Void: _________________ Substitution: _______________________

What do you need to do to follow up? _______________________

every day
-is a-
fresh
START

Breakfast:

Lunch:

Dinner:

Snacks and Drinks:

Exercise:

What went well? _______________________________________________

What can I do better? ___________________________________________

Breakfast:

Lunch:

Dinner:

Snacks and Drinks:

Exercise:

What went well? _______________________________________________________

What can I do better? ___________________________________________________

Breakfast:

Lunch:

Dinner:

Snacks and Drinks:

Exercise:

What went well? _______________________________________________

What can I do better? ___________________________________________

## ▶——— DAY 11   DATE:  ◀

Breakfast:

Lunch:

Dinner:

Snacks and Drinks:

Exercise:

What went well? ________________________________________________

What can I do better? ____________________________________________

## DAY 12   DATE:

Breakfast:

Lunch:

Dinner:

Snacks and Drinks:

Exercise:

What went well? _______________________________________________

What can I do better? ___________________________________________

## DAY 13   DATE:

Breakfast:

Lunch:

Dinner:

Snacks and Drinks:

Exercise:

What went well? ____________________________________________________________

What can I do better? ____________________________________________________________

Breakfast:

Lunch:

Dinner:

Snacks and Drinks:

Exercise:

What went well? ________________________________________________

What can I do better? ___________________________________________

# WEEKLY CHECK-IN

<table>
<tr><td>

**How have I done?**

</td><td>

Date: ______________________

Weight: ______________________

</td></tr>
<tr><td>

**Any takeaways?**

</td><td>

—— Fitness Achievements ——

</td></tr>
</table>

Everybody can have a tough day, and one tough day can send all your good intentions out the window! It's how you approach a tough day that makes all the difference.

One way to prevent disaster happening is to anticipate your tough days and plan for them. Knowing that you have strategies in place before the event will put you in a position to react accordingly and treat a tough day as a tough day - not an excuse to give up!

Brainstorm some strategies for a tough day here:

______________________________________________

______________________________________________

What can you do to follow up? ______________________

______________________________________________

nobody said it was easy

It may not be easy but I know I can cope because _______________________

_______________________________________________________________

_______________________________________________________________

_______________________________________________________________

Breakfast:

Lunch:

Dinner:

Snacks and Drinks:

Exercise:

What went well? ___________________________________________________________

What can I do better? _______________________________________________________

Breakfast:

Lunch:

Dinner:

Snacks and Drinks:

Exercise:

What went well? _______________________________________________

What can I do better? ___________________________________________

Breakfast:

Lunch:

Dinner:

Snacks and Drinks:

Exercise:

What went well? ______________________________________________________________

What can I do better? _________________________________________________________

# DAY 18   DATE:

Breakfast:

Lunch:

Dinner:

Snacks and Drinks:

Exercise:

What went well? ______________________________________________________

What can I do better? _________________________________________________

Breakfast:

Lunch:

Dinner:

Snacks and Drinks:

Exercise:

What went well? _______________________________________________________

What can I do better? ___________________________________________________

# DAY 20  DATE:

Breakfast:

Lunch:

Dinner:

Snacks and Drinks:

Exercise:

What went well? _______________________________________________

What can I do better? __________________________________________

# DAY 21  DATE:

Breakfast:

Lunch:

Dinner:

Snacks and Drinks:

Exercise:

What went well? _______________________________________________

What can I do better? ___________________________________________

How have I done?

Any takeaways?

Date: ___________________________

Weight: _________________________

—— Fitness Achievements ——

What happens when you can't control what you eat and how much you exercise? Perhaps you accept an invitation for dinner at a friend's house, or you go to stay with your parents over the holidays. To be a good guest, you should eat and appreciate the food you are given, within reason.

- You can anticipate. If you are going out for a big dinner, you might eat a more frugal breakfast and lunch.

- You can compensate afterwards, perhaps adding in an extra workout and eating more veg for the next day or two.

How will you cope when you aren't in control?

Just keep swimming

━━━━━━━ DAY 22  DATE:

Breakfast:

Lunch:

Dinner:

Snacks and Drinks:

Exercise:

What went well? _______________________________________________

What can I do better? ___________________________________________

# DAY 23    DATE:

Breakfast:

Lunch:

Dinner:

Snacks and Drinks:

Exercise:

What went well? _______________________________________________________________

What can I do better? __________________________________________________________

**Breakfast:**

**Lunch:**

**Dinner:**

**Snacks and Drinks:**

**Exercise:**

What went well? _______________________________________________

What can I do better? ___________________________________________

## DAY 25  DATE:

Breakfast:

Lunch:

Dinner:

Snacks and Drinks:

Exercise:

What went well? _______________________________________________

What can I do better? ___________________________________________

Breakfast:

Lunch:

Dinner:

Snacks and Drinks:

Exercise:

What went well? ______________________________________________________

What can I do better? __________________________________________________

Breakfast:

Lunch:

Dinner:

Snacks and Drinks:

Exercise:

What went well? ___________________________________________________

What can I do better? _______________________________________________

◄———————— DAY 28  DATE: ————————►

Breakfast:

Lunch:

Dinner:

Snacks and Drinks:

Exercise:

What went well? _______________________________________________________

What can I do better? ___________________________________________________

# WEEKLY CHECK-IN

<table>
<tr><td>

**How have I done?**

</td><td>

Date: ___________________________

Weight: ___________________________

—— Fitness Achievements ——

</td></tr>
<tr><td>

**Any takeaways?**

</td><td></td></tr>
</table>

It is a fact of life that when we change our behaviour - and it starts to show - other people will come out of the woodwork and tell us that we are doing it all wrong!

You may be having a lot of success by counting your carbs. They will warn you to count calories instead! You are wrong and they are right. It is all too easy to get distracted and veer off track.

This would be a good time to look back over the last 4 weeks and decide how you are going to approach the next few weeks.

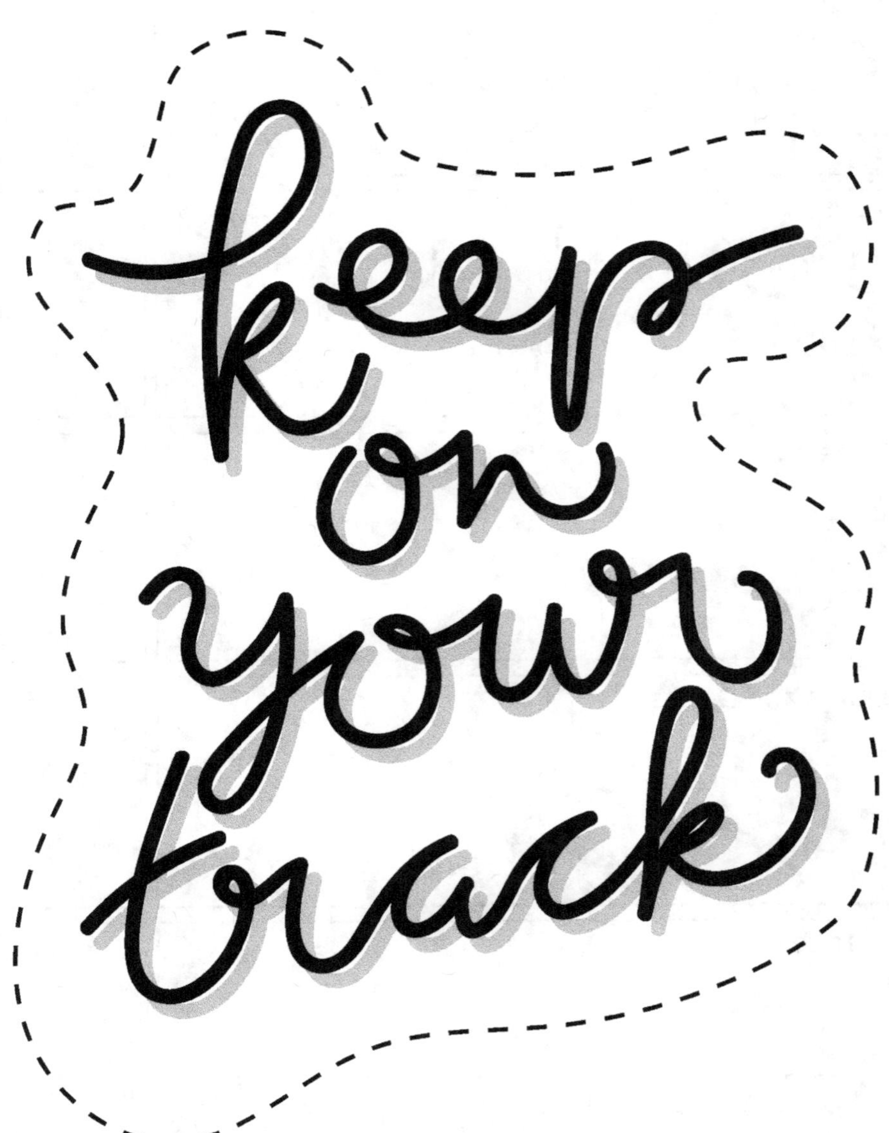
keep on your track

◀━━━━━━━ DAY 29  DATE:  ━━━━━━━▶

Breakfast:

Lunch:

Dinner:

Snacks and Drinks:

Exercise:

What went well? _______________________________________________________________

What can I do better? _________________________________________________________

Breakfast:

Lunch:

Dinner:

Snacks and Drinks:

Exercise:

What went well? _______________________________________________________

What can I do better? ___________________________________________________

# DAY 31   DATE:

Breakfast:

Lunch:

Dinner:

Snacks and Drinks:

Exercise:

What went well? _______________________________________________________

What can I do better? ___________________________________________________

Breakfast:

Lunch:

Dinner:

Snacks and Drinks:

Exercise:

What went well? ____________________________________________________________

What can I do better? ________________________________________________________

Breakfast:

Lunch:

Dinner:

Snacks and Drinks:

Exercise:

What went well? _______________________________________________________________

What can I do better? __________________________________________________________

## DAY 34   DATE:

Breakfast:

Lunch:

Dinner:

Snacks and Drinks:

Exercise:

What went well? ______________________________________________________

What can I do better? _________________________________________________

Breakfast:

Lunch:

Dinner:

Snacks and Drinks:

Exercise:

What went well? ________________________________________________

What can I do better? ____________________________________________

# WEEKLY CHECK-IN

**How have I done?**

**Any takeaways?**

Date: ___________________________

Weight: _________________________

—— Fitness Achievements ——

Do you beat yourself up? Are you more critical of yourself than you would be of a family member or friend?

Or do you congratulate yourself for every positive achievement, and every small step that you take towards your goals? How about looking back over the last week or two and coming up with some reasons to congratulate yourself, here and now!

Action: _______________________________________________________

Action: _______________________________________________________

Action: _______________________________________________________

How can you reward yourself today? ___________________________

___________________________________________________________

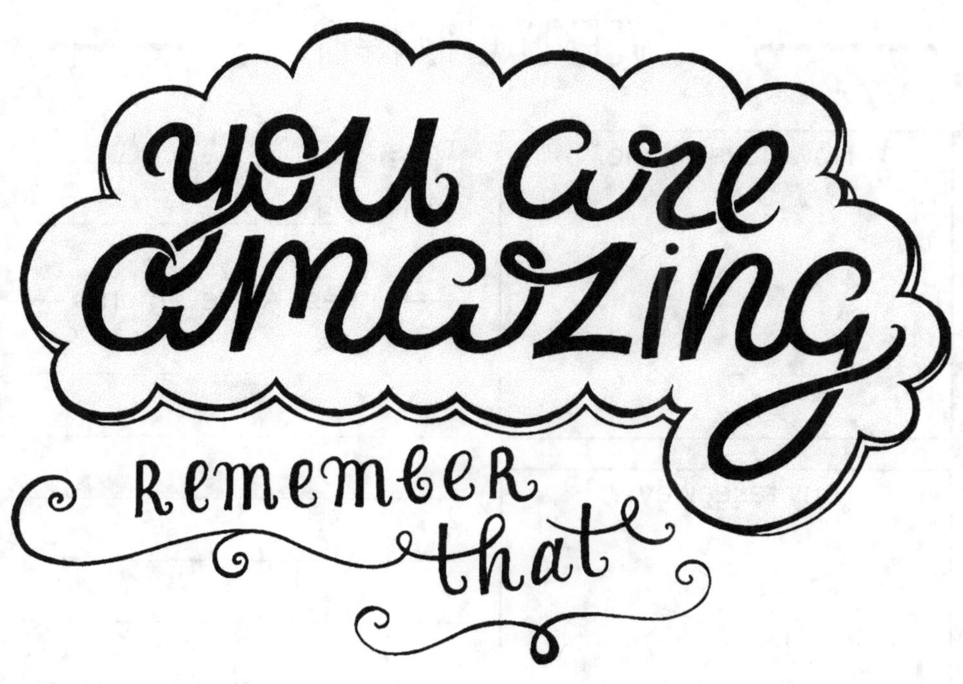



Time to big yourself up a bit! Write down some ways that you are amazing here. Enjoy yourself!

---

＞———————— DAY 36  DATE:

Breakfast:

Lunch:

Dinner:

Snacks and Drinks:

Exercise:

What went well? ___________________________________________________________

What can I do better? ______________________________________________________

## DAY 37   DATE:

Breakfast:

Lunch:

Dinner:

Snacks and Drinks:

Exercise:

What went well? _______________________________________________

What can I do better? ___________________________________________

## DAY 38   DATE:

Breakfast:

Lunch:

Dinner:

Snacks and Drinks:

Exercise:

What went well? _______________________________________________

What can I do better? ___________________________________________

Breakfast:

Lunch:

Dinner:

Snacks and Drinks:

Exercise:

What went well? _________________________________________________________________

What can I do better? _____________________________________________________________

Breakfast:

Lunch:

Dinner:

Snacks and Drinks:

Exercise:

What went well? _______________________________________________________

What can I do better? _________________________________________________

════ DAY 41   DATE:

Breakfast:

Lunch:

Dinner:

Snacks and Drinks:

Exercise:

What went well? _______________________________________________

What can I do better? ___________________________________________

Breakfast:

Lunch:

Dinner:

Snacks and Drinks:

Exercise:

What went well? ___________________________________________________

What can I do better? ________________________________________________

# WEEKLY CHECK-IN

How have I done?

Any takeaways?

Date: _______________________

Weight: _______________________

—— Fitness Achievements ——

On what criteria do you judge yourself? Do you judge yourself on looks, fitness, wealth, or perhaps the number of friends you have? Did you grow up believing you had to be a certain way? Are you comparing yourself to family members, friends, colleagues or social media "influencers" and celebrities? Why? Why do you need to judge yourself or compare yourself at all?

be
your own
kind of
beautiful

# DAY 43   DATE:

Breakfast:

Lunch:

Dinner:

Snacks and Drinks:

Exercise:

What went well? _______________________________________________

What can I do better? __________________________________________

＝＝＝＝＝ DAY 44   DATE:

Breakfast:

Lunch:

Dinner:

Snacks and Drinks:

Exercise:

What went well? ________________________________________________________________

What can I do better? ___________________________________________________________

Breakfast:

Lunch:

Dinner:

Snacks and Drinks:

Exercise:

What went well? _______________________________________________________________

What can I do better? ___________________________________________________________

◄───── DAY 46   DATE:  ────►

Breakfast:

Lunch:

Dinner:

Snacks and Drinks:

Exercise:

What went well? ____________________________________________

What can I do better? ______________________________________

Breakfast:

Lunch:

Dinner:

Snacks and Drinks:

Exercise:

What went well? _______________________________________________________

What can I do better? ___________________________________________________

# DAY 48   DATE:

**Breakfast:**

**Lunch:**

**Dinner:**

**Snacks and Drinks:**

**Exercise:**

What went well? ______________________________________________

What can I do better? _________________________________________

Breakfast:

Lunch:

Dinner:

Snacks and Drinks:

Exercise:

What went well? __________________________________________________________________

What can I do better? ____________________________________________________________

# WEEKLY CHECK-IN

How have I done?

Any takeaways?

Date: _______________________________

Weight: _____________________________

—— Fitness Achievements ——

You are now just over half way through this 90 day tracker. Have you kept tracking relentlessly, even on days when you have slipped up? Or have you, like most people, gone off the rails some days and "forgotten" to record the results?

If you slip up now and then, does it matter over the longer term? No! What matters is giving up.

Do you remember why you started this tracking journey? Remind yourself here:

FALL DOWN
seven
times
GET UP
eight

◀━━━━━ DAY 50  DATE:  ━━━━▶

Breakfast:

Lunch:

Dinner:

Snacks and Drinks:

Exercise:

What went well? ........................................................

What can I do better? ...................................................

Breakfast:

Lunch:

Dinner:

Snacks and Drinks:

Exercise:

What went well? _______________________________________________

What can I do better? _______________________________________________

Breakfast:

Lunch:

Dinner:

Snacks and Drinks:

Exercise:

What went well? ________________________________________________

What can I do better? ____________________________________________

# DAY 53   DATE:

Breakfast:

Lunch:

Dinner:

Snacks and Drinks:

Exercise:

What went well? ______________________________________________________________

What can I do better? _________________________________________________________

## DAY 54   DATE:

Breakfast:

Lunch:

Dinner:

Snacks and Drinks:

Exercise:

What went well? ________________________________________________

What can I do better? ____________________________________________

# DAY 55   DATE:

Breakfast:

Lunch:

Dinner:

Snacks and Drinks:

Exercise:

What went well? _______________________________________________

What can I do better? _______________________________________________

Breakfast:

Lunch:

Dinner:

Snacks and Drinks:

Exercise:

What went well? _______________________________________________________

What can I do better? ___________________________________________________

# WEEKLY CHECK-IN

**How have I done?**

**Any takeaways?**

Date: _______________________________

Weight: _____________________________

—— Fitness Achievements ——

Can you get through just one more day?

If you have a long journey to make, it can be tempting to give up before you have seen it through to the very end. But once you have made it half way, the journey becomes less daunting. You are now well passed half way and on the home stretch! Just keep going, one day at a time, and soon you will have reached your goal.

Tactics for making it through one more day:

Reasons not to quit:

______________________________________________

______________________________________________

______________________________________________

______________________________________________

______________________________________________

◄━━━━━━ DAY 57  DATE:

Breakfast:

Lunch:

Dinner:

Snacks and Drinks:

Exercise:

What went well? ___________________________________________

What can I do better? _______________________________________

Breakfast:

Lunch:

Dinner:

Snacks and Drinks:

Exercise:

What went well? _______________________________________________________

What can I do better? ___________________________________________________

# DAY 59  DATE:

Breakfast:

Lunch:

Dinner:

Snacks and Drinks:

Exercise:

What went well? _______________________________________________________

What can I do better? ___________________________________________________

Breakfast:

Lunch:

Dinner:

Snacks and Drinks:

Exercise:

What went well? ________________________________________________

What can I do better? ___________________________________________

Breakfast:

Lunch:

Dinner:

Snacks and Drinks:

Exercise:

What went well? ______________________________________________________

What can I do better? __________________________________________________

Breakfast:

Lunch:

Dinner:

Snacks and Drinks:

Exercise:

What went well? _______________________________________________________

What can I do better? ___________________________________________________

Breakfast:

Lunch:

Dinner:

Snacks and Drinks:

Exercise:

What went well? _______________________________________________________

What can I do better? ___________________________________________________

# WEEKLY CHECK-IN

| How have I done? |
| :-- |
|  |

Date: _______________________________

Weight: _____________________________

—— Fitness Achievements ——

| Any takeaways? |
| :-- |
|  |

Have you been feeling deprived? If you start to feel like you are missing out it is all too easy to allow yourself *"just* one small bite" or "a small drink, *just* for tonight".

Or perhaps this week it has been easier to stay home rather than put on your workout clothes and hit the gym - *"just* this once".

Oh no! It's time for a reset! Don't let the *"justs"* derail you!

Your reasons to keep going:

HELLO
new day

Breakfast:

Lunch:

Dinner:

Snacks and Drinks:

Exercise:

What went well? ______________________________________________________________

What can I do better? __________________________________________________________

Breakfast:

Lunch:

Dinner:

Snacks and Drinks:

Exercise:

What went well? _______________________________________________________

What can I do better? ___________________________________________________

Breakfast:

Lunch:

Dinner:

Snacks and Drinks:

Exercise:

What went well? _______________________________________________________

What can I do better? ___________________________________________________

◄———————— DAY 67  DATE:                    ———————◄

Breakfast:

Lunch:

Dinner:

Snacks and Drinks:

Exercise:

What went well? ___________________________________________________

What can I do better? ______________________________________________

## DAY 68   DATE:

Breakfast:

Lunch:

Dinner:

Snacks and Drinks:

Exercise:

What went well? ________________________________________________

What can I do better? ____________________________________________

## DAY 69  DATE:

Breakfast:

Lunch:

Dinner:

Snacks and Drinks:

Exercise:

What went well? ____________________________________________

What can I do better? ______________________________________

Breakfast:

Lunch:

Dinner:

Snacks and Drinks:

Exercise:

What went well? _______________________________________________

What can I do better? ___________________________________________

# WEEKLY CHECK-IN

How have I done?

Any takeaways?

Date: ________________________________

Weight: ______________________________

—— Fitness Achievements ——

Sometimes we can get so stuck into a routine - particularly if we are tracking it - that we fail to grow and improve. This week, challenge yourself to do something better, faster or stronger!

Record your ideas here:

Dare

-TO-

Grow

Breakfast:

Lunch:

Dinner:

Snacks and Drinks:

Exercise:

What went well? _______________________________________________________

What can I do better? __________________________________________________

◀━━━━━ DAY 72  DATE:  ━━━━▶

Breakfast:

Lunch:

Dinner:

Snacks and Drinks:

Exercise:

What went well? _______________________________________________

What can I do better? _________________________________________

◄———————— DAY 73  DATE: ————►

Breakfast:

Lunch:

Dinner:

Snacks and Drinks:

Exercise:

What went well? _______________________________________________________

What can I do better? __________________________________________________

◄━━━━━ DAY 74  DATE:  ━━━━►

Breakfast:

Lunch:

Dinner:

Snacks and Drinks:

Exercise:

What went well? ________________________________________________

What can I do better? ____________________________________________

Breakfast:

Lunch:

Dinner:

Snacks and Drinks:

Exercise:

What went well? _______________________________________________

What can I do better? ___________________________________________

Breakfast:

Lunch:

Dinner:

Snacks and Drinks:

Exercise:

What went well? ___________________________________________________________

What can I do better? _______________________________________________________

⟶ DAY 77  DATE:

Breakfast:

Lunch:

Dinner:

Snacks and Drinks:

Exercise:

What went well? _______________________________________________

What can I do better? ___________________________________________

How have I done?

Any takeaways?

Date: _______________________

Weight: _______________________

—— Fitness Achievements ——

The Japanese philosophy of Kaizen, or "constant and never-ending improvement", suggests that nothing is ever perfect and that there is always room for  refinement. It also suggests that each tiny incremental improvement builds on previous tiny improvements, so that step by tiny step we can reach our goals.

What tiny improvements can you make this week?

MAKE A NEW COMMITMENT
# EVERY DAY!

Breakfast:

Lunch:

Dinner:

Snacks and Drinks:

Exercise:

What went well? _______________________________________________

What can I do better? ___________________________________________

Breakfast:

Lunch:

Dinner:

Snacks and Drinks:

Exercise:

What went well? ________________________________________

What can I do better? ____________________________________

Breakfast:

Lunch:

Dinner:

Snacks and Drinks:

Exercise:

What went well? ______________________________________________________________

What can I do better? __________________________________________________________

Breakfast:

Lunch:

Dinner:

Snacks and Drinks:

Exercise:

What went well? _______________________________________________

What can I do better? ___________________________________________

Breakfast:

Lunch:

Dinner:

Snacks and Drinks:

Exercise:

What went well? ______________________________________________________________

What can I do better? _________________________________________________________

Breakfast:

Lunch:

Dinner:

Snacks and Drinks:

Exercise:

What went well? _______________________________________________________

What can I do better? ___________________________________________________

◀━━━━━━ DAY 84   DATE:

Breakfast:

Lunch:

Dinner:

Snacks and Drinks:

Exercise:

What went well?

What can I do better?

# WEEKLY CHECK-IN

How have I done?

Any takeaways?

Date: ___________________________

Weight: _________________________

—— Fitness Achievements ——

Almost there! There are just a few more days to go until the final check-in at the end of this 90 day tracker, so make sure that they are good ones!

This might be a good time to make arrangements for a reward at the end of the 90 days. Jot down your notes here!

IT'S A
new
day

Breakfast:

Lunch:

Dinner:

Snacks and Drinks:

Exercise:

What went well? _______________________________________________________

What can I do better? ___________________________________________________

◄———— DAY 86   DATE:

Breakfast:

Lunch:

Dinner:

Snacks and Drinks:

Exercise:

What went well? _______________________________________________________

What can I do better? _________________________________________________

◄━━━━━━━ DAY 87   DATE: ━━━━━◄

Breakfast:

Lunch:

Dinner:

Snacks and Drinks:

Exercise:

What went well? _________________________________________________

What can I do better? _____________________________________________

◄■———— DAY 88  DATE:                    ■———■

Breakfast:

Lunch:

Dinner:

Snacks and Drinks:

Exercise:

What went well? ________________________________________________

What can I do better? ___________________________________________

# DAY 89   DATE:

Breakfast:

Lunch:

Dinner:

Snacks and Drinks:

Exercise:

What went well? _______________________________________________

What can I do better? ___________________________________________

Breakfast:

Lunch:

Dinner:

Snacks and Drinks:

Exercise:

What went well? ________________________________________________

What can I do better? ________________________________________________

# FINAL CHECK-IN

| | Date started | Date completed | Change |
|---|---|---|---|
| Weight | | | |
| Chest | | | |
| Waist | | | |
| Hips | | | |
| Thigh | | | |
| Calf | | | |
| Fitness | | | |
| | | | |
| | | | |
| | | | |
| | | | |

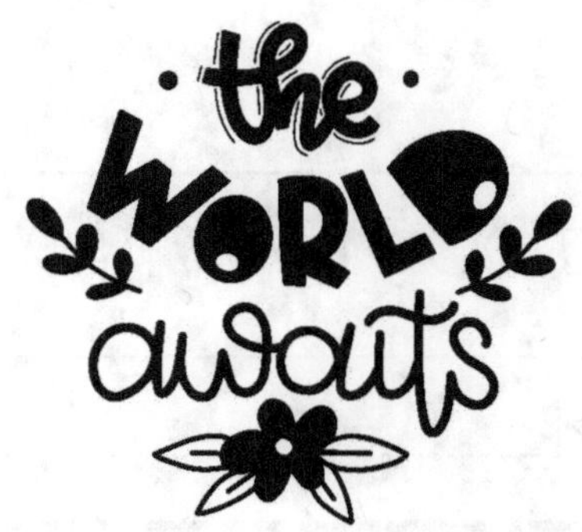

If you have a good day, record the page number here so that you can find it easily, and then repeat it!

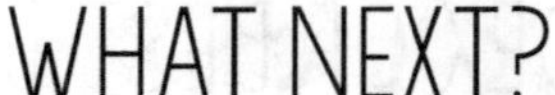

# WHAT NEXT?

Now that you've tracked for 90 days, what next? Did you achieve your goals? Do you need to "rinse and repeat" for another 90 days? If so, what will you do the same and what will you change?

make
your
days
count ♡